Includes a 21-Day Meal Plan & 35 Healthy Snack Options

Eat to Wealth

YOUR SIMPLE GUIDE TO EATING INTELLIGENTLY

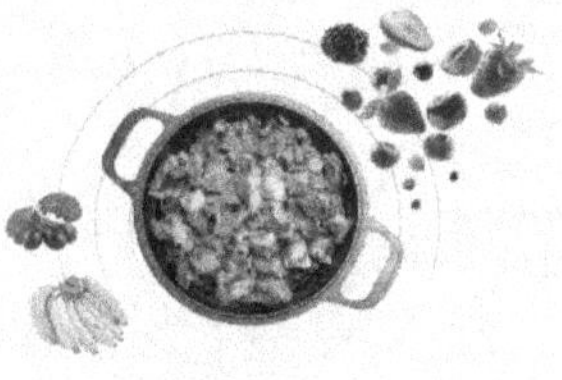

DR JESUPELUMI ADENIHUN

Make this Book a Gift

From:

To:

Date:

Eat to Wealth

YOUR SIMPLE GUIDE TO EATING INTELLIGENTLY

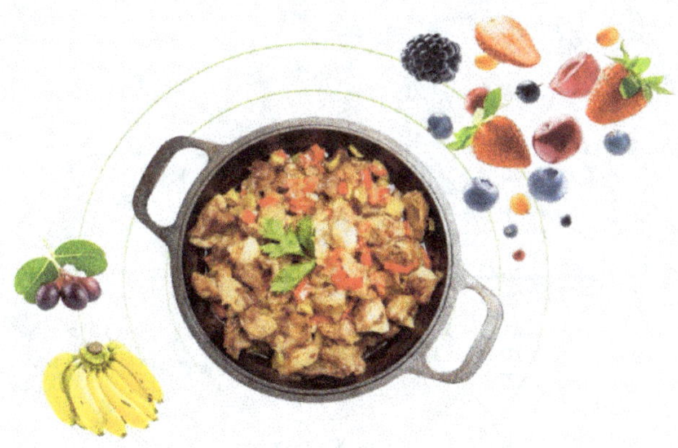

DR JESUPELUMI ADENIHUN

CONTENTS

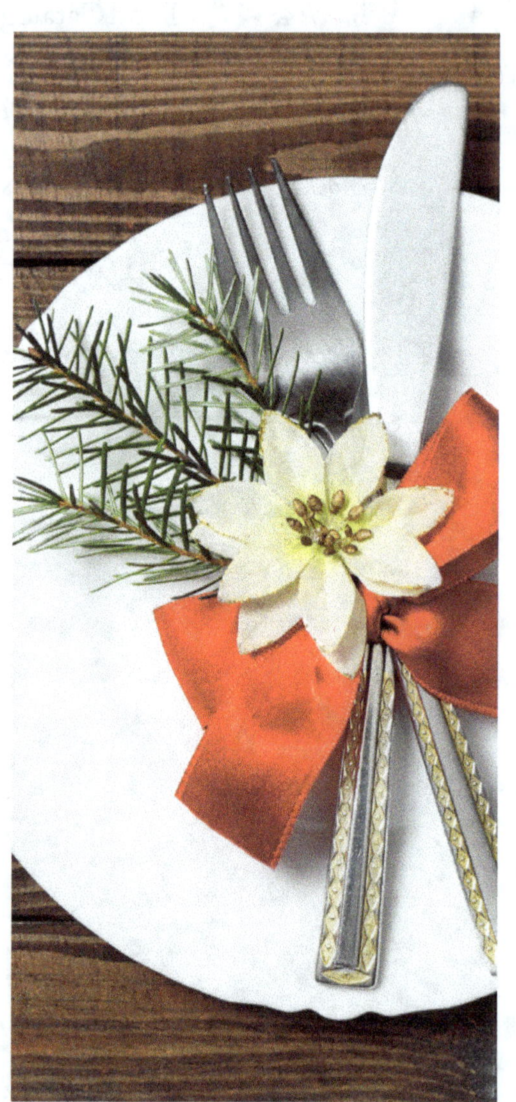

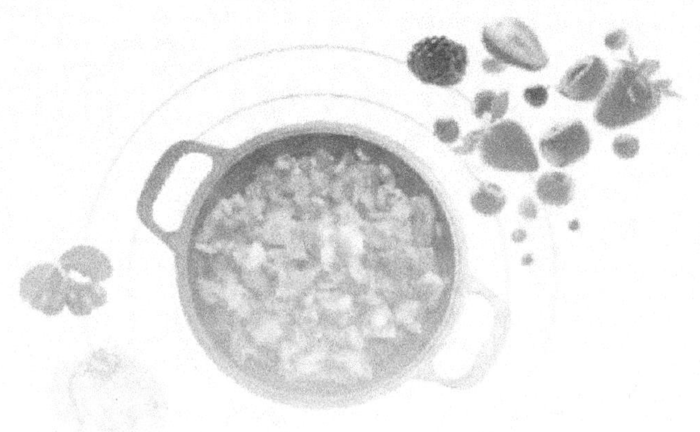

DEDICATION

This book is dedicated to you who have made a decision to live your best life and eat to wealth!

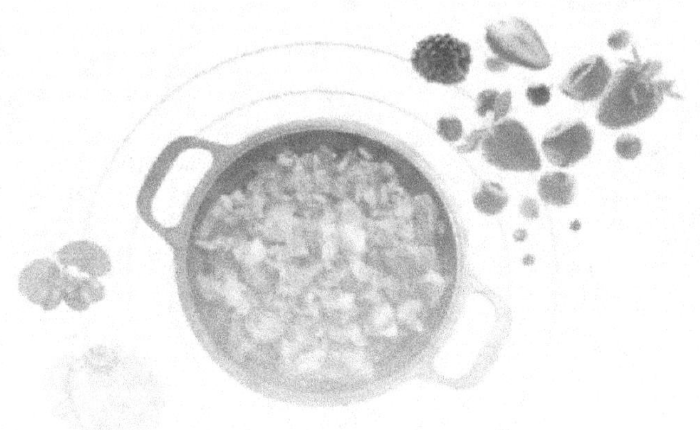

ACKNOWLEDGEMENT

To my King, Defender, Promoter, Chief Igniter and Grace supplier - God, I am indeed grateful for the grace and privilege to have written this book.

I am also thankful for the immense support received from my parents - Dcn Adebayo & Dcns Adebunmi Adenihun, my brother, IfeOluwa Adenihun, my sisters - The Handmaidens, and my entire extended family for ever being a strong pillar of support.

I will not fail to recognize my teachers and mentors; Dr. Folu Olatona, Dr. Babayemi Osinaike, Dr. Olayemi O. Dawodu, Dr. Detolu Adewole, Dr. Mario Adelaja, Dr. Olori-Boye Ajayi, who have constantly cheered me on and offered guidance to me on my journey.

To the amazing contributors to this work - Dr. Ikechukwu Chukwu, my excellent and global standard designer, Okpata Chiderah, my editor, Dr. Minka.Ndifon, my proofreader thank you so much! To my co-founders who would not hold back in seeing me excel, Victor Emaye and Ifedamola Adefisoye, it's such a pleasure having you both as my partners. Thank you!

To my church family who have played an integral part in the person I am today, a big thank you to members of Yaba Baptist Church and The New Church for cheering me on.

Mr. Mike Ogunwale and his entire team, my publisher who worked tirelessly in seeing 'Eat to Wealth' come to life, Thank you for birthing this book!

I am also grateful to you holding this copy whose engagement and commitment to a healthier life inspires my work. Your trust in the knowledge you are about to receive is truly valued." Thank you so much!

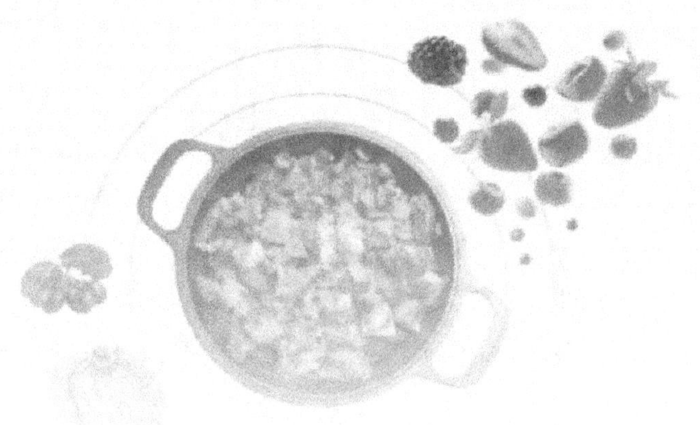

FOREWORD

In a world where wellness and healthy lifestyle practices have become an indispensable pursuit, Dr. Jesupelumi Adenihun has emerged as a guiding light, illuminating the path toward healthy living and disease prevention through the power of nutrition. As a well-learned Medical Doctor, her wisdom and passion have combined to create a beacon of knowledge in the realm of preventive healthcare.

Eat to Wealth is not merely a collection of insights; it is a roadmap to transformative health and well-being and as a member of a globally recognized nutrition body, she brings a holistic perspective that bridges the gap between medical science and the everyday choices that shape our lives.

What sets this book apart is its actionable approach backed by the understanding of the interplay between food and health and then translating this into simple and practical advice. Through these pages, you will find not just information, but a personalized and modifiable companion on your journey toward optimal health.

As a thought leader, two-time author, and co-founder of a pioneering health tech company, Dr. Adenihun's influence extends beyond the written word and shows her unwavering dedication to empowering individuals to take charge of their health destinies.

Eat to Wealth is an invitation to embrace the healing power of food, chart a course toward vitality, and cultivate a lifestyle that is sustainable and thrives in its entirety.

Associate Professor, Dr. Folu Olatona.

Consultant Public Health Physician, Nutritionist, and wellness expert.

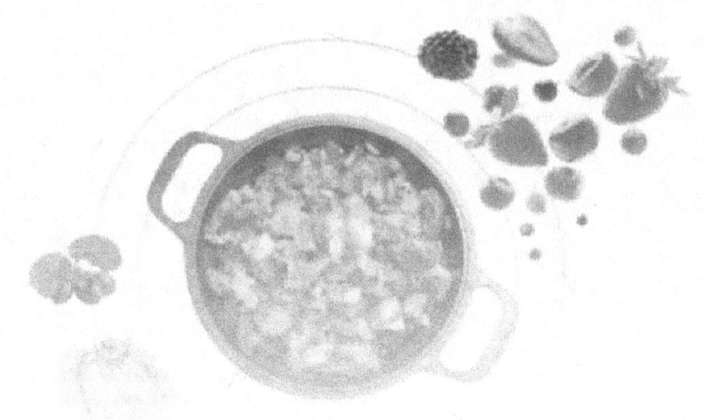

INTRODUCTION

As humans creating our world, we have constantly gone through ideations and birthed innovations that have made our lives comfortable. With each passing day, there is news of a system, software, or product with the potential to improve our lives toward a more desirable future.

We live in a world of endless possibilities where the paradigms through which people live spur them into greater expressions of themselves. Many great men and women have lived through the sands of time. Some lived full lives, others had lonely periods, and some suffered illnesses that shortened their years and a decent number did not even get to see how far their innovations impacted the world.

A common ground we share as humans is the appreciation of good health. Globally, there has been an alarming rise of diseases like diabetes, stroke, heart-related disease, cancers, and so on, all of which research has linked the development of these diseases to the foods we consume. To then ignore how we eat would be to ignore our health, slide into unhealthy states and eventually deprive the world of the best gifts of ourselves, for only when we are healthy can we optimally create and innovate.

Eating to Wealth is not your regular diet book but has been put together to help you see how to take charge of your eating patterns, creatively make your food work for you, and understand the simplicity of eating. There is an art to eating. There is also the knowledge required to know the right things to eat as well. Although simple, the tips and insights shared here would usher you into your journey to wealth - not just for you but for all those that matter to you.

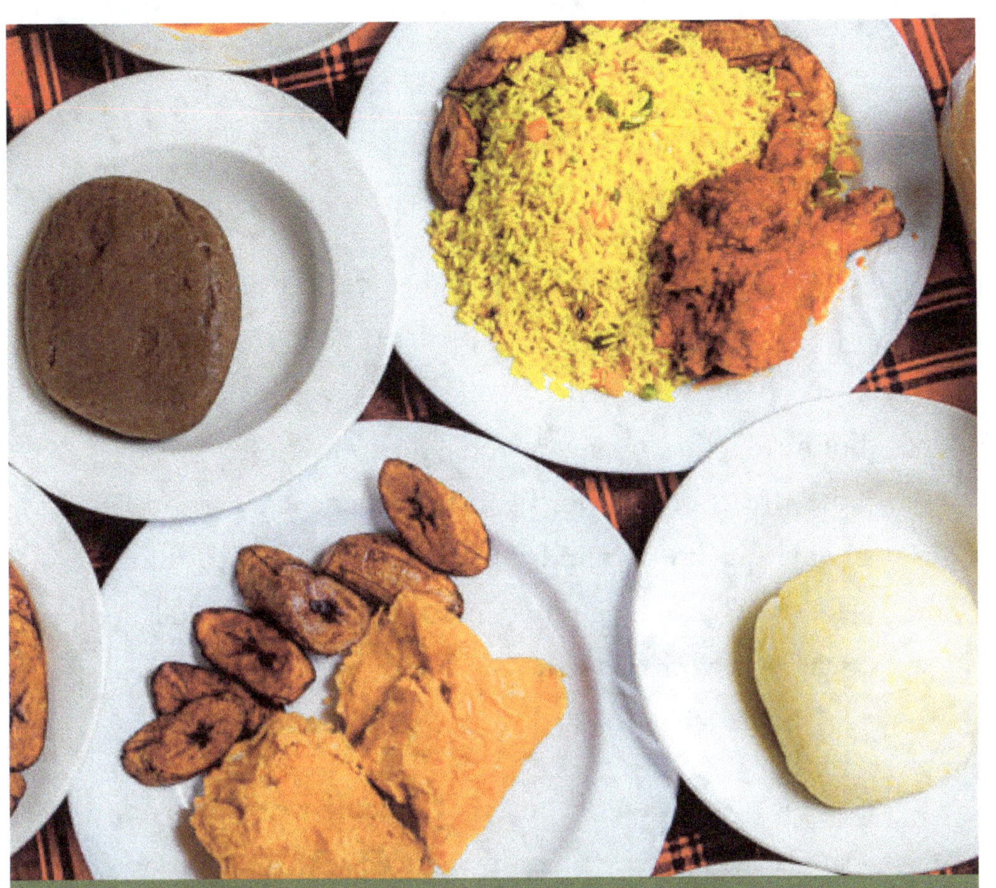

EATING

What exactly is it that we do when we eat? Having encountered this word repeatedly, one would wonder if there is more to it than taking in food. However, as I sit to write, the effects of this word and the experiences around it come quickly to mind. I am also compelled to think about what eating really means. Is eating a skill, a scientific work to be studied, or is there a school to go to learn to eat right and to do so with enthusiasm?

In the programs and courses of learning we embark on, subject matters are often introduced with a definition. Words mean different things to us and sometimes, we forget or lose the meaning of the words we come across hence, the need to get reminders. The definition of **eating** would serve as a reminder and perhaps realign your perspective on what the otherwise common concept is.

What is Eating?

1.   According to the Merriam-Webster Dictionary, Eating means to take in through the mouth as food: ingest, chew, and swallow in turn.

2.   Wikipedia defines Eating (also known as consuming) as the ingestion of food, typically to provide a heterotrophic[a] organism with energy and to allow for growth.

A second look at the definitions will leave room to absorb their meanings, particularly the definition by Merriam Webster which shows that to eating, there is first an **'action'**, then a **'process'**, and finally, an **'outcome or goal'**.

It is, therefore good to state that;

Eating is an action that initiates a process to provide an outcome.

Eating ⇨ Process ⇨ Outcome

This shows that every time food is eaten, different processes are being initiated, resulting in compounding outcomes that may either turn out to be beneficial or harmful. All of this is, however, based on the first action, eating. To change the outcome would require that changes be made to the first step, *eating*, which boils down to the steps leading to what you eat and the constituents of your meal.

Think about it, what is the best meal you have had in the last seventy-two (72) hours? What is it that intrigued you about that particular meal? Was it the taste, the person who made it, where it was eaten, the event or moments shared around the meal (like Nigerians would say - party jollof rice[b]), or had it just been a while since you had something that tasty?

We all experience the act of eating differently and for different reasons - for strength, other times for pleasure, comfort, social connections, celebrations, and much more. While all these reasons are valid, the most important reason to always hold on to is to *eat for health*.

Benjamin Franklin once said:

'*We eat to live and not live to eat*',

and another by Bethenny Frenkel reads:

"*Your diet is a bank account. Good food choices are good investments.*"

Ultimately, you are either investing in good or bad health by how you eat.

As you continue in this book, I trust you will become more accountable for your eating decisions. Beyond becoming accountable, the aim is to enjoy the processes and steps involved rather than see them as a chore. Let me state here that the intention of this book is not to put you in a 'diet' box, seeing we almost all get discouraged at the mere mention of the word *diet*.

One thing this book will do is help build within you an internal operating system that is continuously and sustainably geared toward eating healthy. I also encourage you to read it more than once to grasp and stay in touch with everything communicated.

For many, eating healthy is the goal. *Healthy* meaning eating foods good enough to meet the body's nutritional requirements for the different phases of life. However, when a good number of people hear the term 'healthy eating', they imagine eating only leafy greens like spinach for the rest of their lives which is not so. You will soon see here that with the vast array of foods nature has made available, you can choose from different options to achieve your goal of healthy eating even when there are specific health needs.

If you would take home one point from this chapter, it should be that *healthy living is a lifetime course and not a one-time goal*. It is one you should continuously improve on as you get better equipped with the knowledge and tools required to do so. You must, however, be *willing* and *patient* with yourself to make adjustments gradually.

Now let's see how well you understand.

Questions for you.

1. What is eating?

2. What are the most typical or frequent reasons you eat for?

---

a. **Heterotrophic** - a living thing that gets nutrients from food and plants).

b. **Party Jollof** is a colorful rice meal that Nigerians and Ghanaians argue over who makes it better. For the party jollof, it has a peculiar woody/smokey and delicious taste. See to try it if you've never had it.

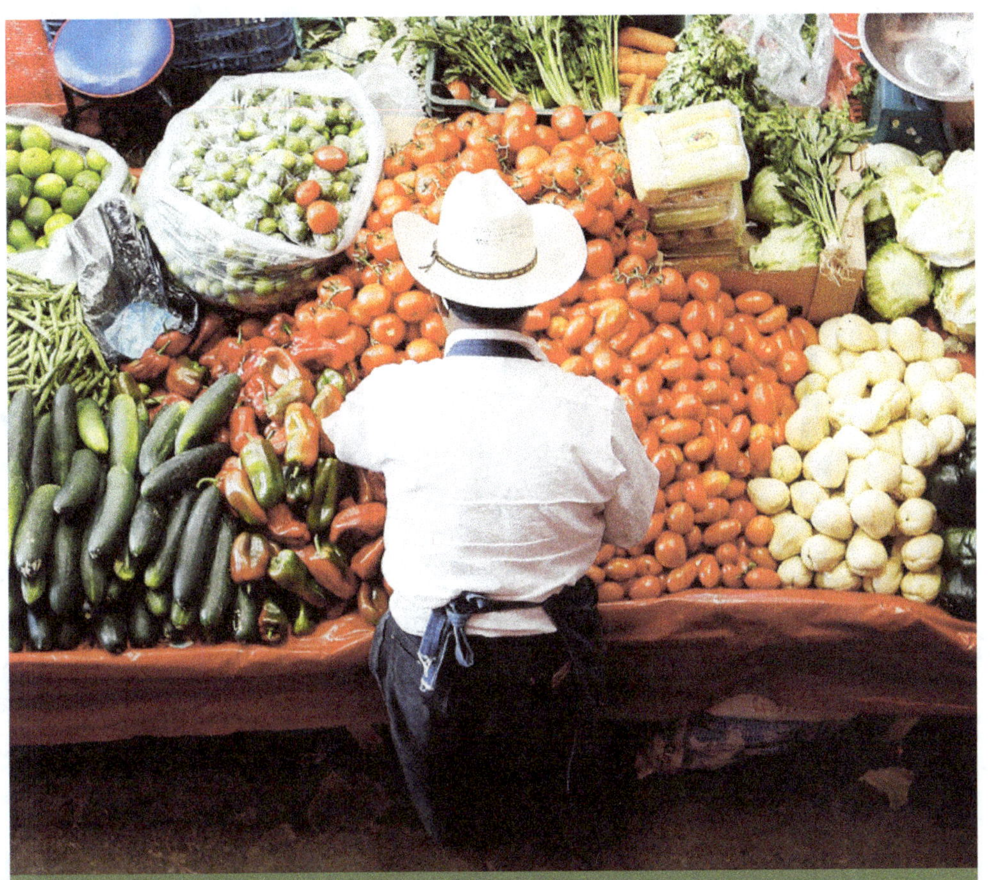

BLOCK 2
CULTURE, WORK
AND FEEDING

CULTURE

Ever wondered why you eat the way you do? Or do you find that you are constantly and repeatedly consuming the same food type - rice, potatoes, bread, etcetera? While there is absolutely nothing wrong with eating those meals, the danger lies in the tendency to get bored with eating, coast into a state of unhealthy eating, and then lose one's appetite altogether. A typical scenario is a diabetic[c] who has been wrongly subjected to feeding on unripe plantain or beans only, in their varied form. Such persons eventually see eating as a task rather than something they should enjoy or benefit from.

No doubt, there are times we experience seasonal love for certain foods and eat those till our taste buds get weary of them before picking on a new food interest. Again, the beauty of eating as seen in subsequent chapters is that there is a wide array of foods to choose from per food group and geographical location. The world also, being a global village, coupled with technological advancements and innovations in the agro sector has made room for agricultural exchanges. It has now become possible to cultivate foods within controlled environments and maintain the integrity of their nutritional content, and effect on the human body.

In considering the foods available across different food groups, you would come to see that the nutrients required in the body are provided by the combination of different food items and that the factors that affect weight gain or loss have to do with - the quantity of food eaten, quality (referring to the nutritional content), level of physical activity, hormonal changes, stress levels, phase of life (reproductive or nursing) and chronological age.

Back to the question posed earlier, figured out the reason behind your eating pattern yet?

Ponder on it for a moment......

Just as the case is in other areas of life, our eating patterns are largely influenced by what was modeled in our developmental phase as children as well as environmental influences.

The cultural differences existing across societies also serve as pointers to why specific groups are more predisposed to certain diseases than others seeing that people within a cultural setting are more inclined to eat similar foods. For some, it could be taking mainly fries, oil-dense meals, or overly processed foods. Thankfully, culture, being a way of life, can be deliberately changed and improved on. The critical thing to know is your culture of eating should be redefined in line with the health outcomes you desire.

A typical example is the southwestern part of Nigeria, often known to have large amounts of pepper or palm oil in their meals. Intrinsically, there is nothing wrong with taking these - pepper or palm oil. The issue arises when they are eaten in large amounts, which poses a risk for stomach ulcers or increased cholesterol levels predisposing to heart-related issues. In this case, the eating behavior around these foods can then be adjusted or significantly reduced. This is one example; there is the need to take a look at what you may have culturally imbibed that is not suitable for you or your health.

WORK

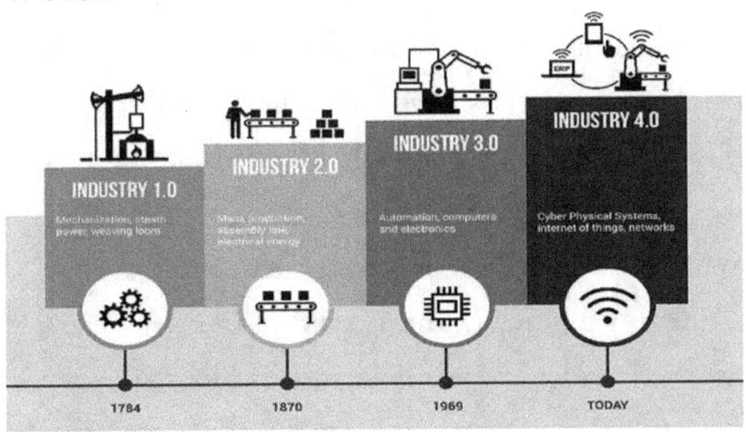

Work is man's gift. The industrial revolutions that have taken place across centuries have revealed man's innate abilities to create for himself a continuing better world. From heavy-duty machines to small-sized devices capable of doing so much and now robots, there is no end to these innovations. It is imperative that as we create and innovate, we must adapt.

Data has it that the number of people who now work from home has tripled, with statistics on that increasing rapidly, owing largely to the effect of the COVID-19 pandemic. The changes in work patterns are not entirely new developments. Before the 2020 pandemic, reports showed a decline in the rate of physical activity as people had become less active at the workplace either remotely or from a physical location. What used to be predominantly defined as work in terms of gathering, hunting, and farming manually has been replaced by technological solutions, which in themselves have improved our living conditions generally. Only we are now sitting more, bending over screens, and working from one position for hours. It has even happened that a person's job could be used to predict what type of disease(s) they are likely to be affected by. The question then lies in identifying the appropriate eating pattern for the work types we find ourselves in.

There is no one-size-fits-all, especially when it comes to nutrition and health. However, there are slight and deliberate modifications that can be made to accommodate the healthy lifestyle you hope to achieve.

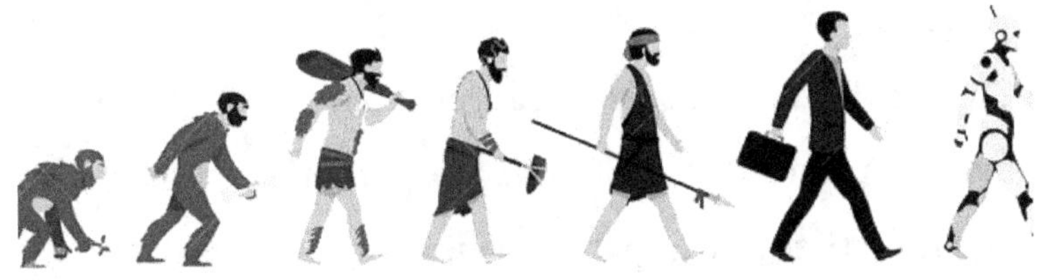

Image illustrating the change in the working pattern of man.

The first step to change is the awareness of what needs to be changed. Again, this would require some reflection as there is the need to recondition your mind on what your body needs to function effectively as an individual, especially as you transit across the different phases of your life since eating has a habitual process to it. How you eat is a habit, and because different energy levels are required for the roles we take up or the phases we go through, it is important to take into consideration the quantity of food being consumed (a highly physically active person or athlete will typically consume larger portions of food), the quality (e.g., nursing mothers or mentally active people are advised to take in nutrient-dense[d] meals), the type of meal (e.g., starchy or proteinous foods) the time it is being consumed (certain meals are better consumed earlier on in the day than late at night to aid digestion and proper utilization of the meal) and the effect it has on you.

The body is great at communicating, so instances like feeling very heavy after a meal, especially if in one position on a repeated basis, may indicate the need to adjust the quantity or type of food. Another instance is those who experience feelings of bloatedness or passage of loose stools after taking certain foods, e.g., milk. Commonly referred to as lactose intolerance. In this situation, it is often advised to find alternatives, such as plant-based milk instead of milk from animals. It is also good to note that certain foods provide a laxative effect after eating them as they aid bowel movement. A major category of this includes vegetables, which contain fiber, are nutritious, and are still very good to eat.

In today's world, despite the fact that people sit a lot often, we are still always in a hurry. This applies especially to those resident in highly urbanized cities. Always hurrying to make a call, get something done, move somewhere, or grab a meal. There is a lot of activity, and everything seems to be in a heightened state of a rush. This state, the fast-paced mode of living, turns out to be counteractive to our health. When eating is done in a rush, there is an increased likelihood of overeating, the digestion process is hindered which can lead to uncomfortable feelings afterward and in some cases, a feeling of dissatisfaction. The digestive system has its control centre in the brain, so the brain is also involved in notifying when one is full. However, hurried eating can affect this process. What then is the way out of this?

Regarding eating, it is not only what you eat that matters but how you eat, as already mentioned. A look into one of the *'how to's'* of eating is when you eat, eat **intentionally**.

What is intentional eating, you may say?

Beyond the deliberate effort of the meal type or quality being taken, intentional eating has a lot of **mindfulness** involved. To be mindful of what you eat is to engage fully in the experience of the meal you are having, i.e Take an active meal break with no distractions - no tv, phone scrolling, working while eating, or the other ways we multitask while eating. Yes, this sounds like a crazy idea and can be quite a challenging thing to adjust to particularly because a good number of us have cultivated the habit of eating and watching a movie, reading or working. It's okay to have company when you eat, but when eating alone, be in the moment of your meal and do so when seated calmly. What happens is you begin to experience the full flavors of your food and even get to observe what goes through your mind as you eat. As much as possible, avoid standing to eat or eating in a hurry. To do this may require deliberately setting aside breaks to eat. However, forming a habit requires gradual change and intentionality, which may involve cues like setting alarms to grab a meal. The overall aim of this is to ensure that quality meals are taken mindfully.

A vast majority of people spend about a third of their day at work. You then observe that factors like 'time availability', the location of work, access to good foods or fresh produce, and even having to handle important aspects of life like school, family, and other areas sometimes make eating healthy a task.

Before moving to the next chapter, take note of how the work you do influences your feeding pattern and think of possible solutions that will help achieve the eating pattern you desire.

When time is a major hindrance, it may be the cue for you to outsource meals, delegate the meal preparation if that option is available for you or prepare meals in bulk so you take them when needed. Access to healthy food options at the workplace may sometimes be a challenge which is why having homemade meals packed to work is often encouraged. However, in the absence of this, the option is to source for cafeterias that prepare relatively good meals or order from restaurants you are familiar with.

The understanding with this is to take note of the little improvements you can make and progressively build on them. Do not aim to be perfect in achieving what your definition of healthy eating is at the onset; instead, be happy to take steps that move you closer to that goal.

Questions:

1.   Are there unhealthy cultural patterns you have observed around your meal consumption?

2.   If yes, what is it you can do to change that?

3.   What eating habits have you developed around work?

4.   What can you do to improve on it?

5.   Are there things you think you need to start eating less of or more of based on your current phase of life?

c.   A diabetic is someone who has a disease called diabetes. Diabetes is a condition where the body has high levels of blood glucose, also known as blood sugar, and can pose lots of problems in the body.

d.   Nutrient-dense meals are meals that are rich in nutrients. The American Heart Association refers to Nutrient-dense as foods that are rich in vitamins, minerals, and other nutrients important for health, without too much saturated fat, added sugars, and sodium. These include whole grains, fruits, vegetables, nuts, legumes, seafood, eggs, etc.

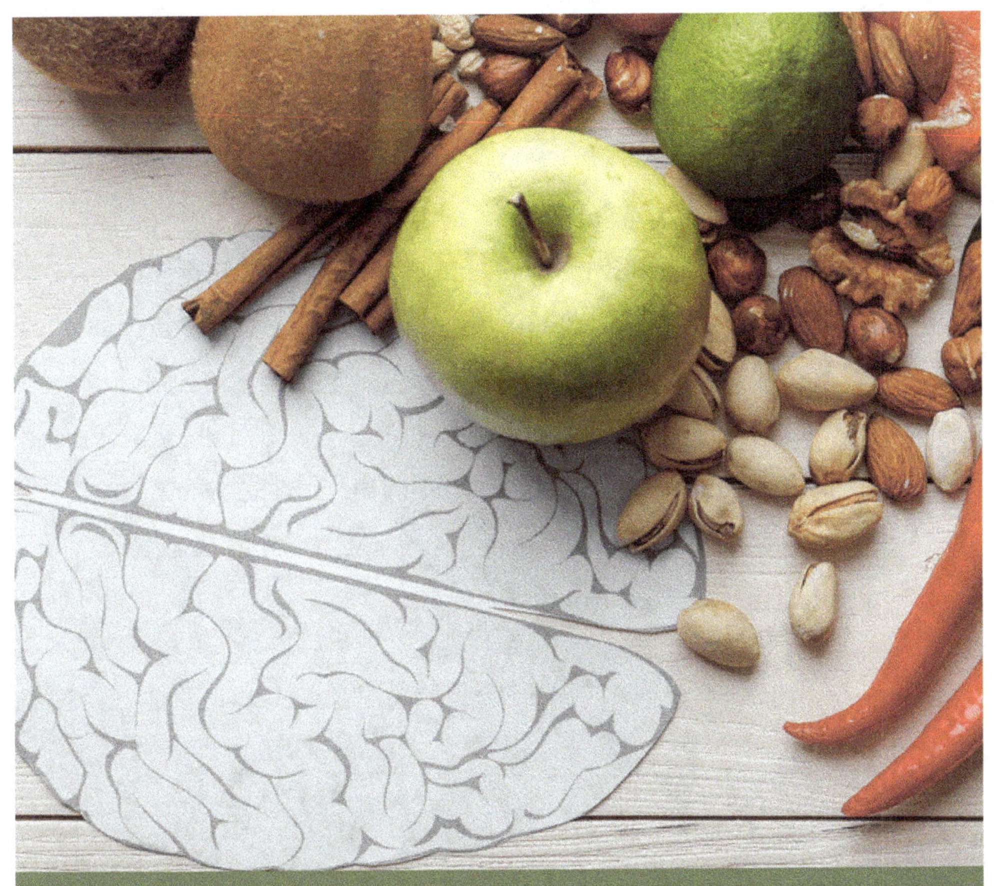

23

Much research has gone and is still being carried out on why people eat the way they do and how food affects the body. When we talk about psychology, it refers to behavior towards eating in this case. As highlighted in the previous chapter, behavior towards food and eating can be unlearned and relearned.

Take a look at these two plates:

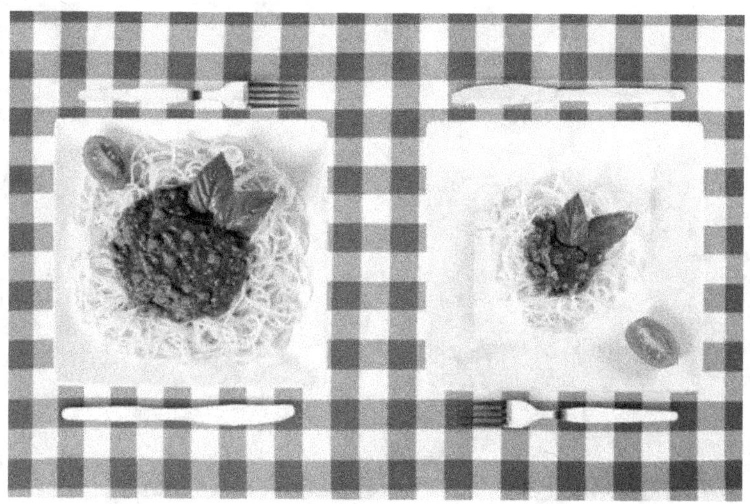

Ever happened that you ate a meal that seemed small but actually ended up filling you? Or you dished out what looked like a lot on a plate only to end up consuming it all? I bet you have had either of those experiences. Perhaps eating is a mind thing after all!

If that is the case, making plate sizes work to your advantage is something worth doing. Want to reduce the amount of food you eat? Use smaller plates (*and resist the urge to go for second portions when you are done eating, particularly if you are working on losing weight*). Want to take in more to gain weight or build mass? See to use bigger plates if that would help you eat more (as that has been shown to help eat more to put on weight). Again, there is no 'one size fits all' when it comes to eating, but these are general principles that apply. There is the need to also understand the body type you possess and see what works for you based on what you intend to achieve.

Media and a lot of food marketing have had quite some influence on our food choices and consumption patterns. For example, a drink in a 500ml pack goes for a certain amount, and then the 1500ml (1.5L) size of it goes for a very discounted amount. The tendency is to go for the bigger size because that looks like a fair deal which is not bad in itself, only that unhealthy foods are now cheap and abundant, thus increasing their rate of consumption. An advert depicting certain foods or drinks as heroic objects also influence food choices. The aim of this is to help you see how these factors affect our consumption patterns so you can better be in charge and be conscious of making healthy choices.

Food cravings, defined as an intense desire to consume a particular food (or type of food) that is difficult to resist, have been shown to occur frequently in most of the population. While it may be okay to have days where cravings are satisfied, grab that ice cream, full cheeseburger, a large bowl of food with extra sauce, and so on. Having cravings repeatedly has also been alluded to as a symptom of stress.

The American Psychological Association has defined stress as a normal reaction to everyday pressures, which can become unhealthy when it upsets your day-to-day functioning. Every one of us has encountered stress in one way or the other. The issue with being in a consistent state of stress is the body releases certain hormones, which can result in overeating, increased fat storage, and then weight gain. This is also the reason why certain people engage in numerous practices to lose weight but still find out they aren't shedding any. The stress hormones released counteract their weight loss strategies hence, the need to identify and look at their stress levels.

Back to cravings, it happens to the vast majority of us. Sometimes, there's the craving to settle for something sweet after a really long day at work, a heartbreak or emotional trauma, or an unpleasant occurrence. That is the stress effect. To curb and manage cravings, a few tips that have been shown to help are highlighted below:

- Identify the cause of repeated stress and del with it in the best way you can. Seek professional help if you need to.

- Be mindful of your cravings and ask yourself questions like 'Am I famished or just stressed?'Don' be in a hurry to grab your cravings.

- Prepare your snacks ahead - Decide on what it is you would snack on if you have to. You would later see in this book healthy snack options to have but there still remains a need to practice portion control.

- Eat whole foods. There is a lesser likelihood of having constant cravings when you eat foods that are minimally processed.

- Make use of natural appetite suppressants. Research has shown that certain foods or herbs act as natural suppressants, an example being ginger. What ginger does is it increases the feeling of fullness when taken and can also help with weight loss. Asides from using it as a spice in your meals, you can have it as tea, add it to your water or chew some before you eat.

Those are a few things you can make use of to deal with cravings or overeating as a result of stress.

For humor, consider asking women with kids about their cravings during pregnancy, you would be surprised at the things they craved. To sum this up, eating is learned, and what is repeatedly depicted to you as right or good is what the mind accepts; therefore, everything should be reviewed from the lens of the health benefits.

Questions

1. Am I easily influenced by what I see in the media about food?

2. When it comes to eating, what habits have I noticed I consistently exhibit that may not contribute to my healthy living?

3. Do I have cravings, what do I often crave, and what triggers my cravings?

4. How can I start to change all this?

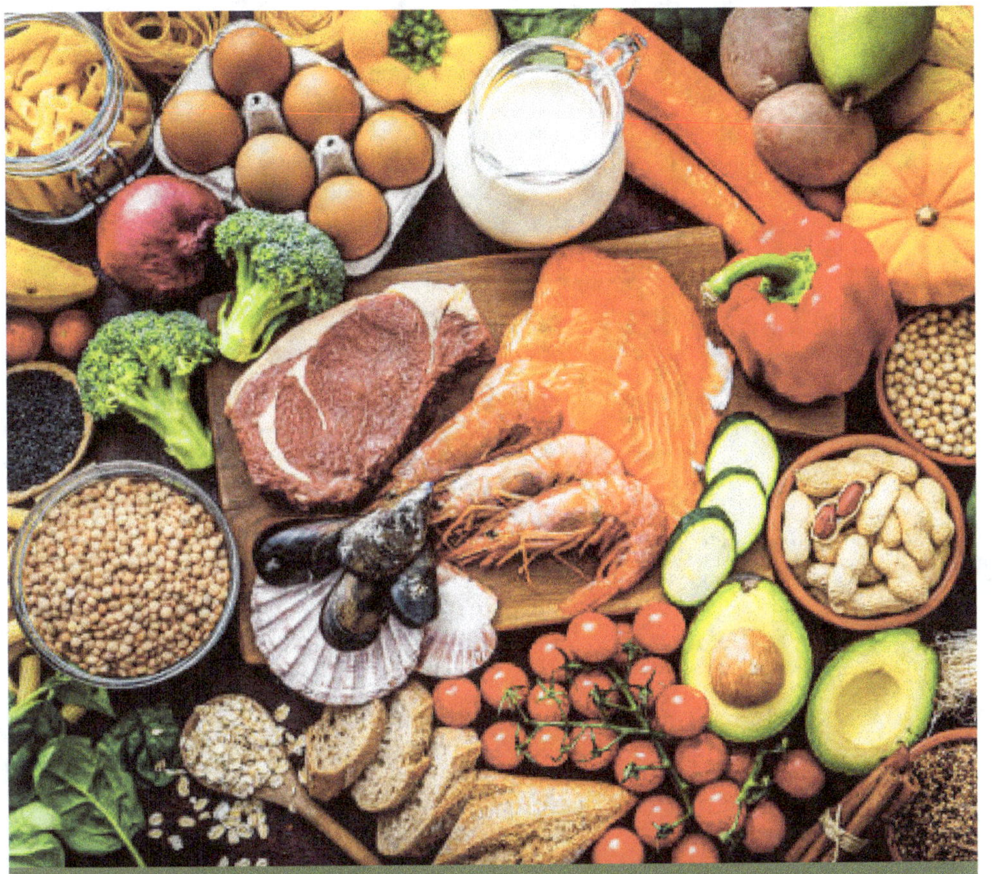

BLOCK 4

FOOD
CATALOG

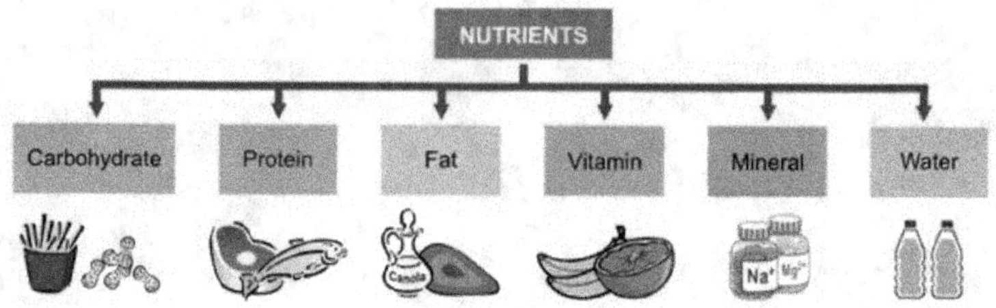

The image above showing the six classes of food serves as a reminder of what makes up a balanced diet. (Simply put, a balanced diet is a meal that contains the food nutrients the body requires).

Now, whether one decides to go vegan, keto, or maintain a current eating pattern, there are numerous options to have as further expanded.

FOOD GROUPS AND THEIR EXAMPLES

There are five known food groups segmented based on the different nutrients they possess. When considering what to eat, see to combine meals across the different food groups. The knowledge of what is under each food group would serve as a guide in your food selections.

1.   **Dairy:** Serves as a good source of protein, calcium, phosphorus, vitamins, and minerals and is derived from milk.

Examples: Milk, yoghurt, fura da nono (dairy product made of millet and fermented milk from Northern Nigeria), wara (milk curds from Southwestern Nigeria), cheese, butter, etc.

Dairy products are not to be consumed in excessive amounts.

2.   **Vegetables**: Rich in vitamins and minerals the body requires in varying amounts. These are further grouped into

•   Bulbs - onions, garlic

•   Stems - celery

- Roots & tubers - carrots, beets, sweet potato,

- Leaves - kale, lettuce,

- Flowers - cauliflower, broccoli,

- Fruits - tomato, cucumber,

- Seeds & pods - peas,

- Fungi - mushrooms.

It is recommended that you have at least 3 servings[e] of vegetables to meet your daily requirements.

Locally grown vegetables in Nigeria- afang leaves, pumpkin leaf (otherwise known as ugu), Lagos spinach (efo shoko), bitter leaves, eggplant leaves, african Spinach (efo tete), waterleaf, wild Lettuce (efo yanrin) Malabar spinach (amunututu), scent leaf and much more.

3. **Fruits:** From the essential vitamins and minerals they contain to their fiber content,

antioxidants[f], and so on, you almost cannot go wrong with fruits.

It is recommended that you have at least 2 servings of fruits[g] daily to meet your body's requirements.

Examples: apple, banana, pineapple, pawpaw, watermelon, star apple (i.e. agbalumo or udara), water/rose apple, sea/tropical almonds(fruit), orange, grapefruit, tamarind(i.e., awin), mango, guava, avocado, cashew apple, tangerine, coconut, soursop (this fruit tastes sweeter than its name), etc.

4. Grains: Great sources of carbohydrates, vitamins, minerals, and fiber, especially when consumed in their whole form. They are also often fortified for added nutritional benefits and constitute a bulk of staple foods eaten. Some examples include rice, wheat, oats, millet, corn, rye, bulgur, quinoa, and sorghum.

5.   **Protein:** This group accounts for foods made from meat, poultry, seafood, peas, lentils, nuts, and seeds. Proteins serve as building blocks for the body. Asides from commonly known animal protein sources, some examples of plant protein include - chia seeds, chickpeas, almond nuts, tofu, lentils, and soybeans.

See below an image illustrating the food groups.

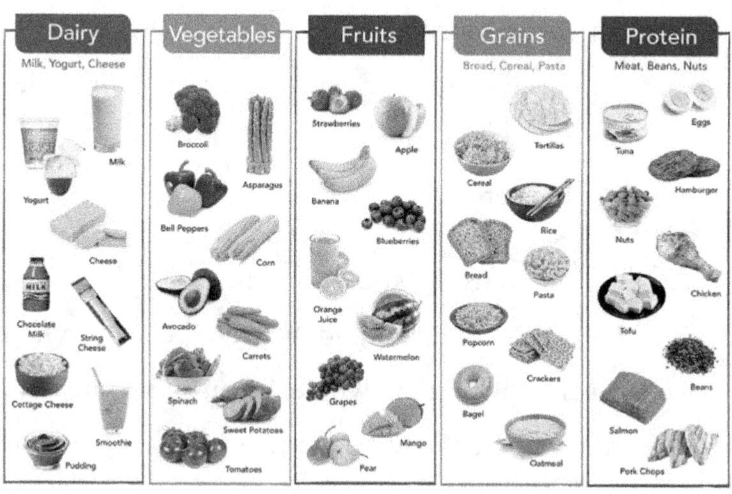

Try a new dish you haven't tried before from the food groups.

g.   A serving of vegetables usually counts as a cup (i.e., about 250mls) of cooked vegetables or two cups of raw leafy vegetables.

f.   Antioxidants are substances in foods that fight harmful radicals which sometimes cause diseases like cancers, heart-related diseases, diabetes, etc)

h.   A serving of fruit is usually whole fruits e.g orange, apple, pear, or a bowl of chopped fruits like watermelon

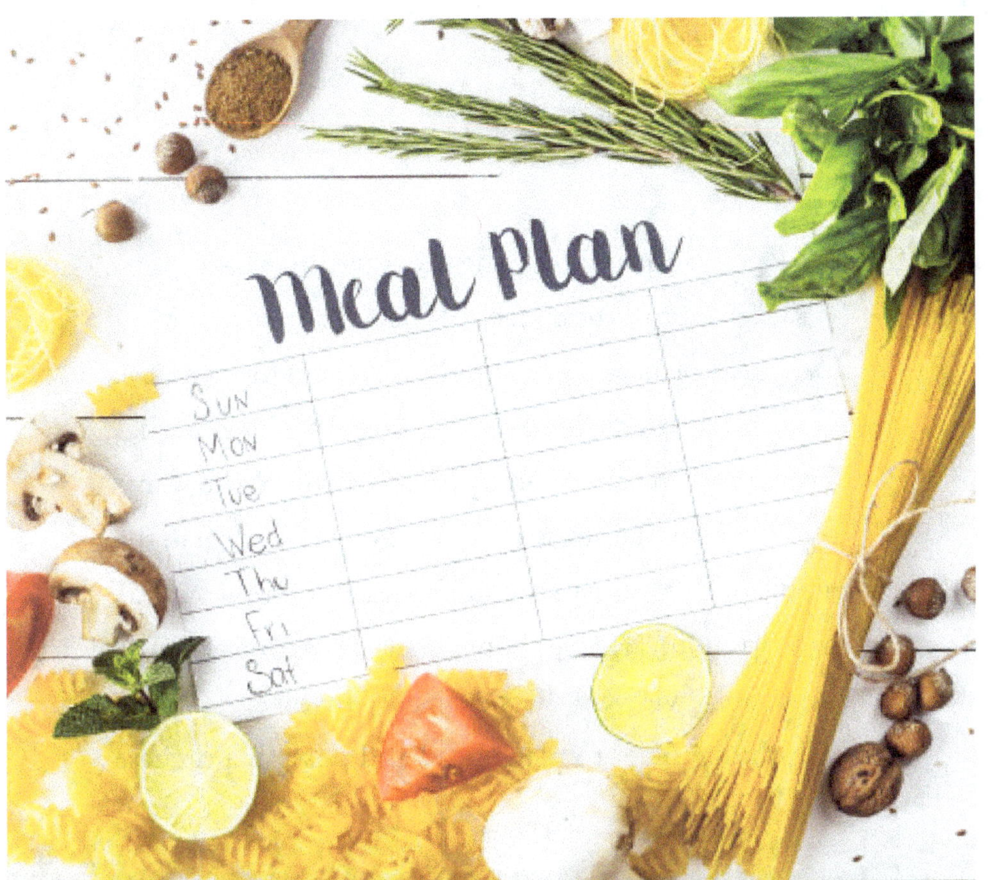

BLOCK 5

TIPS ON USING A MEAL PLAN

At one point or the other, we may have come across the concept of using meal plans. Meal plans are great tools to have. However, the intention is never to keep one in a box. Thinking of what to eat every time can be pretty herculean too. Who wants to go through that stress after a long day at work or in the middle of a very busy schedule? See this more as a guide to help you achieve your goal of eating healthy sustainably with less hassle or cost involved because, with this, you get to plan ahead and possibly purchase food items in bulk.

Meal plans are also tools to enhance better preparation towards having balanced meals. **No single food has it all**. Hence, the need to **merge options** from the different food groups available. A reasonable amount of consideration has been put into the meal plan, ensuring foods are combined across the food groups. The idea is also to avoid getting tired of eating the same things every day and slipping into eating less healthy options out of boredom. The meals suggested here are not ones you must stick to; however, they are much easier to come by, depending on the geographical location you also find yourself in. The adventurous part may be opening up to new food experiences and sampling meals you have never had!

Making or purchasing food items in **bulk** has proven to be a useful tip for many people. Having leftovers isn't a bad idea, either. They could be warmed as next-day meals or whipped into something else. More so, when walking towards health goals, meal plans and preps help keep momentum while figuring out what works best for your body type and schedule.

Regarding meal schedules, it is advised to have meals around the same time of the day as this trains the body on when it should expect to be fed and reduces the tendency to eat randomly. An example of this is setting lunchtime at 2 or 3 pm daily. When this time is kept to regularly, even in instances when one may be carried away by another activity, the body, having been accustomed to lunch at that time, releases hunger cues to indicate meal time. The last meals of the day should typically be taken within two to three hours before bedtime to ensure proper digestion and fewer abdominal upsets. That means for a bedtime of 10 pm, the last meal of the day should be no later than 7 or 8 pm. The earlier, the better.

On sourcing food items, remember to use seasonal foods while they are available. For not-so-common foods, the internet has made it easy to purchase such items. Friends and local communities are also good sources of information when it comes to buying food items. Taking it further is to consider having a mini garden to grow some foods if that interests you.

To close out on this, meal plans happen to simulate the regular plans we make daily. However, the more plans are made, the better the outcomes. When making your own meal plan or deciding on what to eat per day, with the knowledge you have now received of the food groups, it is advised to pick meals across the various food groups. As opposed to having only rice, bread, or pasta, which all belong to the grain food group, ensure to complement them with foods from other groups to make room for a well-balanced meal.

Question

1.   What do you think a meal plan can help you achieve?

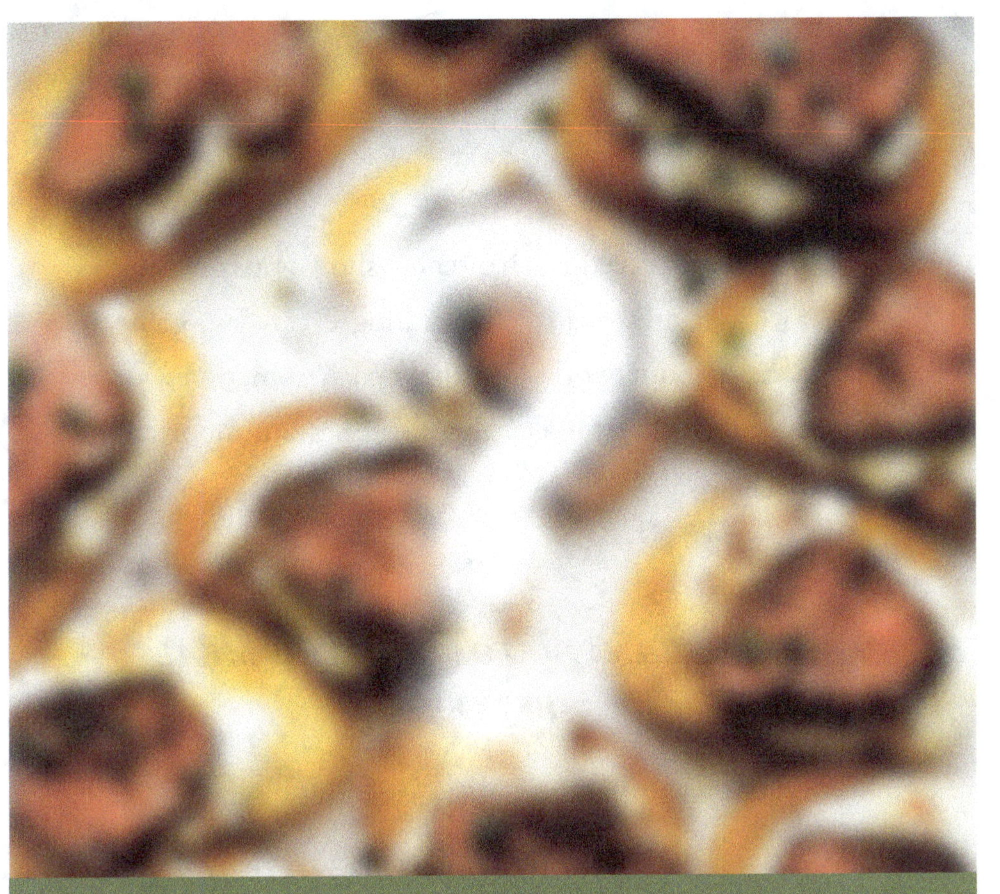

THE BIG QUESTION

The preceding chapter has shown tips on using a meal plan. While eating every day, going about work, skipping meals sometimes, or just feeding off leftovers, there still lies an important question to ask.

*****

WHAT CAN I DO TO MAKE THIS MEAL BETTER?

Yes, it's that simple. Or ask it this way.

HOW CAN I IMPROVE ON THIS MEAL I'M EATING?

Let this be the thought that pops up in your mind every time you settle to eat. What you would realize is the more you ask yourself this question, the more it creates in you the consciousness of eating better.

If this will help, see 'eating better' as a muscle being built or exercised. The more you do it right, the better you get at it. So next time you grab a fork or spoon to eat or decide on a snack, do a quick think on the question - **What can I do to make this meal better?**

The answer may be as simple as grating some carrots and adding chopped cucumbers and cabbage to the intended meal or something more robust like a full vegetable salad. Whatever the case, feel free to enjoy all the experiments you think of!

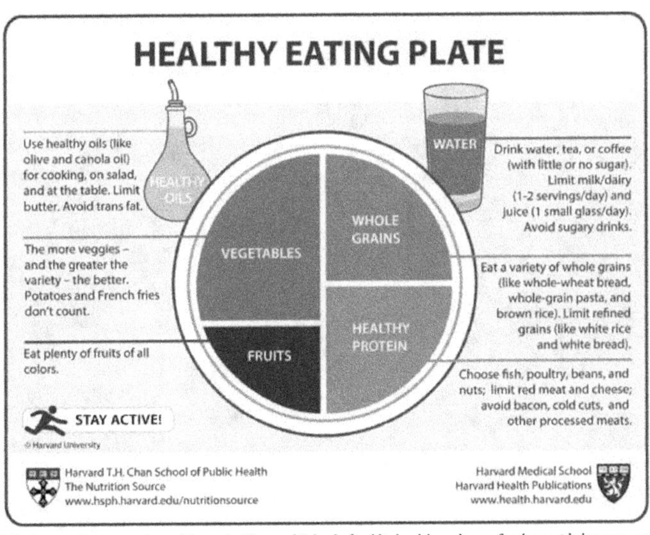

The image above was adapted from the Harvard School of public health and may further guide how you eat.

Question

1. What can you do to make your next meal better?

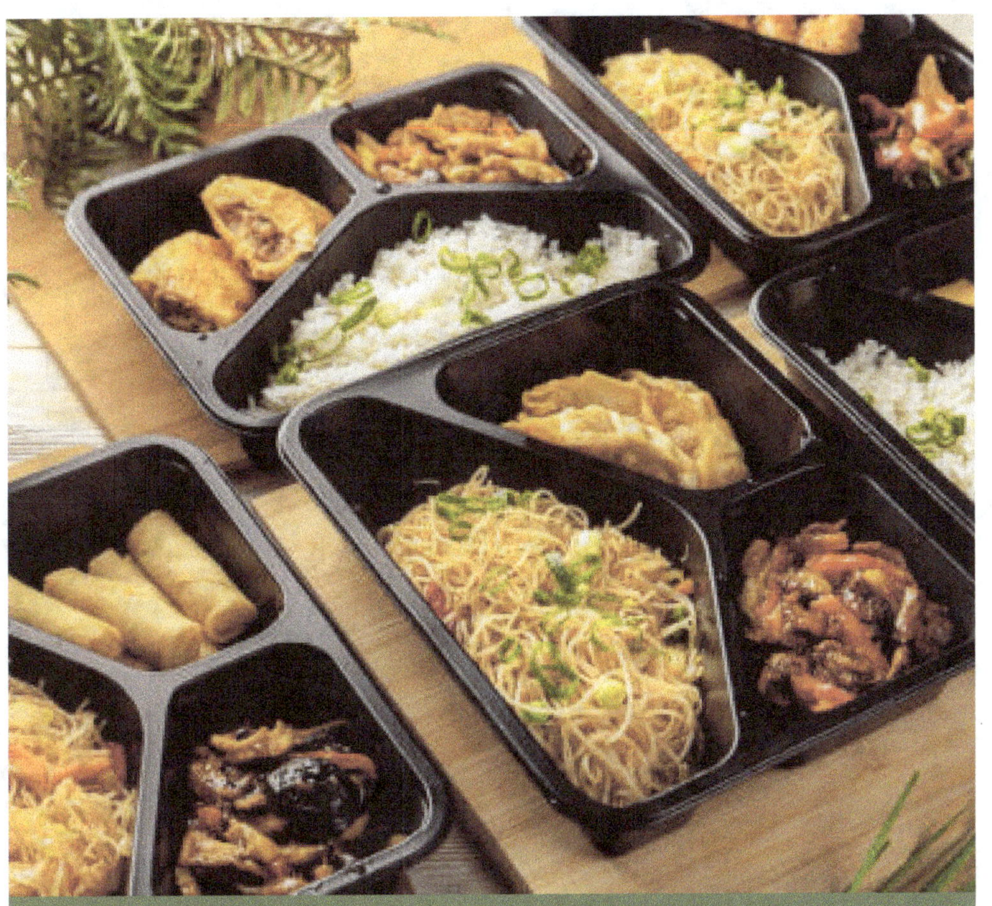

THE 21 DAY MEAL PLAN

Twenty-one (21) days are said to be a good time to build or develop a habit. However, it is not entirely about the duration of time but the consistency that goes into it. At the end of 21 days, it is expected that you have attained a measure of progress with being conscious of what and how it is you are eating. The intention is not to stop after 21 days. Keep at it, redesign if you wish to, or simply shuffle what you already have here. The plan has been split into blocks of seven days. You can check to see how well you are doing after three or seven days or as you deem fit. Remember, the goal is **progression and not immediate perfection**.

DAY 1 - 7

Day	Breakfast	Lunch	Dinner	Snack (optional)
1	Oat porridge, boiled egg, bananas	Pasta, coleslaw, beef/chicken.	Sweet potato, fish sauce.	Watermelon /Pawpaw sliced or diced.
2	Fruit smoothie with nuts	Amala/tuwo/ oatmeal, vegetable soup and fish.	Plantain & egg sauce.	Vegetable salad.
3	Oat porridge, peanut butter, apple	Jollof rice, vegetable salad, chicken/turkey.	Moin moin, vegetable sauce, fish	Popcorn (slightly salted or minimally sweetened)
4	Sandwich, orange juice or whole orange(s)	Porridge beans, fish.	Rice, curry chicken soup	Smoothie

5	Pap and akara. Carrot Sticks	Pasta, sauce, chicken.	Pancake, banana.	Trail mix (see snack list)
6	Moinmoin, Bread, cucumber	Cous cous, veggies, seafood of choice.	Sweet potato, porridge, beef	Zobo drink and cracker
7	Oat, egg, apple.	Eba, afang soup, beef	Fruit salad.	Tiger nut drink.

N.B,

Pap is typically made from maize, sorghum, or millet. It's either prepared alone or mixed with other ingredients, such as ginger, turmeric, etc., for a richer flavour and nutrients.

DAY 8 - 14

Day	Breakfast	Lunch	Dinner	Snack (optional)
8	Bread, egg sauce, carrot sticks	Beans & (sweet) corn porridge	Potatoes, chicken stew, coleslaw	Whole oranges/ Pineapple.
9	Tapioka, milk, coconut shavings.	Rice, chicken. curry sauce and	Parfait (homemade or purchased).	Garden eggs/apple and nut butter or whole nuts.
10	Plantain and egg sauce, carrots.	Rice & beans with fish stew.	Stir-fry noodles, veggies, chicken/ turkey	Guacamole (see snack list)
11	Granola cereal, apple.	Eba/pound ed yam and egusi soup with beef.	Tea/soy drink and Pancakes. Choice fruit	Potato chips and guacamole.

12	Coconut bread, akara, tea, and banana	Wena (masa) and groundnut soup).	Sweet potato, vegetables, fish stew.	Dark-chocolate
13	Yam, egg sauce, orange	Jollof rice, chicken and salad.	Bread and fish stew.	Cake slice and tea/ juice.
14	Plain beans, fish sauce and plantain + vegetables if desired.	Semo/eba baobab soup (kuka)/ okro	Boiled/ fried Irish potato, beef, veggies	Apple and peanut butter.

DAY 15 - 21

Day	Breakfast	Lunch	Dinner	Snack (optional)
15	Cereal choice, apple	Jollof Pasta, sea food or chicken.	Boiled plantain with vegetables and fish.	Carrot cake and tea
16	Yam porridge	Amala/semo/ oatmeal and gbegiri(bean soup) plus ewedu soup.	Quaker oat and fish (grilled or roasted).	Boiled egg
17	Toast bread, milk, and desired	Ofada rice and sauce, beef/goat	Sweet potato, sauce and chicken.	Granola bar
18	Rice and fish sauce. Water melon	Stir fry pasta with chicken.	Fruit/vegetable salad.	Kuli kuli (see snack

19	Oat and egg, Any whole fruit.	Yam and beans.	Bread (toast or plain), spread and tea	Popcorn
20	Banana-based smoothie with nuts	Semo/eba/ wheat with ogbonno soup/ seafood okro and chicken.	Pancakes, milk, or soy drink.	Coconut chips or dried fruits.
21	Desired cereal, and fruit	Go for a buffet, you'll get more ideas too.	After a buffet? A soup or tea and biscuit.	Scotch egg or pie.

More Tips For You

- Snacks are optional and may not be needed especially when whole foods that are rich and satisfying have been taken. There is also the liberty to decide what time of the day to have your snacks.

- In the event you don't have the ingredient for certain foods, you can substitute them with meals within the same food groups. For example, yam can be eaten in the absence of potatoes, other cereals in place of pap, etc.

- Perhaps you get very uncomfortable after taking milk or dairy products- bloatedness, passing loose stools, abdominal pain, etc. Alternatives like skimmed or plant-based milk, e. g almond milk, can be consumed.

- On cooking methods, it is often better to boil or steam than to fry. Fried foods should be eaten occasionally.

- When boiling meals, for example, yam or plantain, the amount of water that is just sufficient to cook those meals is what should be added. Turning out water after cooking is throwing away some of the nutrients.

- Cream in salads is optional. When in use, avoid mixing in too much.

- As a strict vegetarian, animal proteins can be replaced with protein sources like tofu, mushrooms, peas, locust bean, lentils, nuts, seeds, etc.

- Smoothies - make in bulk and preserve in the refrigerator[i]. Nuts and seeds are also good additions to your smoothie. Chia seeds, for example, are a good source of protein and fiber that can be added to your smoothies.

With a meal plan, start with what you have and from where you are at.

It is all about continuous improvements, after all.

See ideas below of five ways to have five common foods.

Yam: Yam porridge, yam & egg sauce, yam & pepper fish sauce, yamarita, yam & pepper soup.

Beans: Beans & sauce, beans porridge and corn, beans & yam, beans & rice, beans & sweet potato.

Potato: Mashed potato, oven-baked potato & sauce, potato & scrambled eggs, potato pepper soup, fries (occasionally).

Rice: Rice & curry sauce, coconut rice, brown rice & sauce, rice & pepper soup, pineapple rice.

Plantain: plantain & vegetables, plantain & egg sauce, plantain porridge, oven-grilled plantain & sauce, plantain & gizzard mix.

Question

1. What problems have you previously encountered when you use a meal plan?

2. Can you make it work for you this time?

---

i.   It has also been said that preserving your smoothies or fruit juices in glass bottles or wares keeps them fresher in comparison to plastic jars or containers. However, you can start with whatever item you have accessible to you and improve on them.

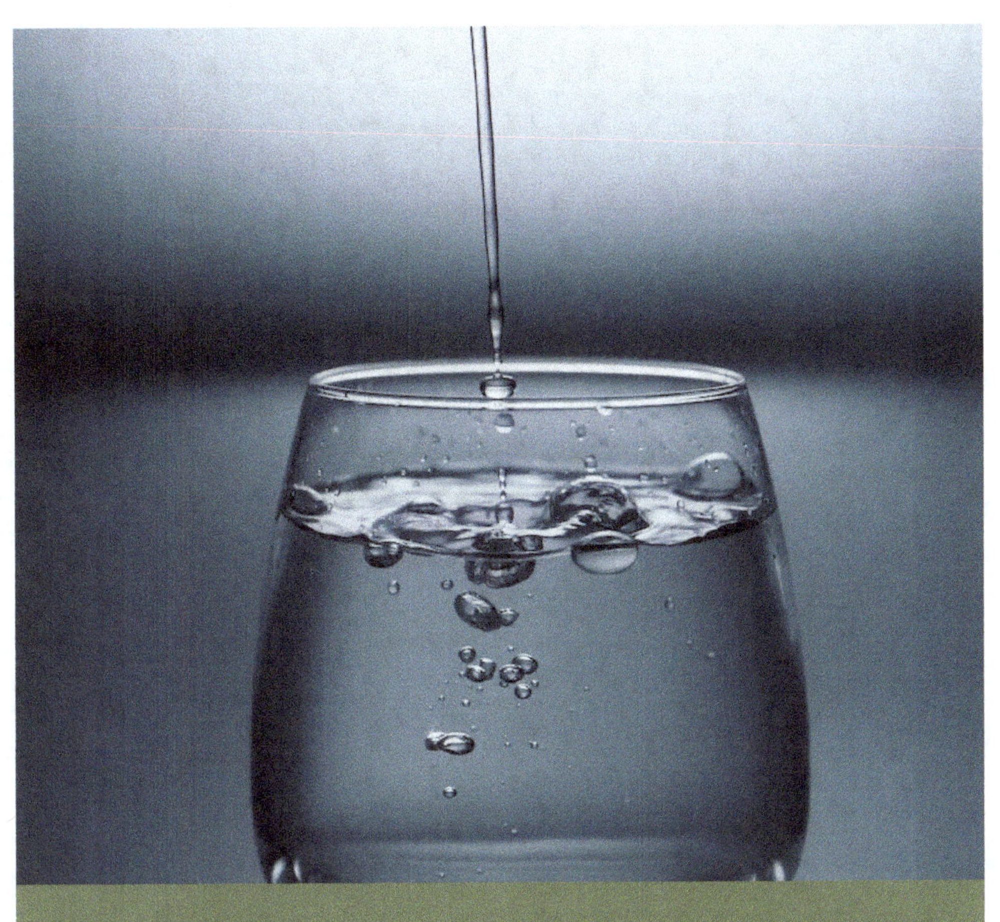

BODY LUBRICANT

Food classes, options, and eating, in general, have been considered. It is time to focus on what brings them together nicely - water. Water is known to be the lubricant of the body, and about 60 - 70% of the body is comprised of water. Hence, the benefits of drinking water or adequate amounts of fluid daily CANNOT be over-emphasized.

Water aids the proper functioning of different organs of the body and has positive effects even on the skin. The benefits of drinking water are enormous, and as a result of physiological mechanisms that have been put in place in the body, our bodies have ways of reminding us when water needs to be taken. For example, thirst is a cue to drink water, and the color of urine is also an indicator of when more water needs to be taken; the darker the urine color, the more water intake is required. However, these should not be relied on alone.

Effectively, water can be taken when you wake, around meal times, and throughout the day having taken into cognisance your daily requirement of about 2 - 3 Liters daily. Asides from water, fruits (particularly juicy ones e.g. watermelon) are also great sources of fluid for the body.

Sometimes, we find that we are addicted or somewhat attached to certain drinks that are not particularly healthy. In this case, it is good to practice the **replacement** principle. What this means is to take something else in place of those drinks. In place of a soda drink, have squeezed fruit juices, a less sugary drink, or natural drinks like tiger nut and others you get to come across. Quite a number of drinks are being made now with little or no additives or sugar in them, and they still taste so good. Some can even be made at home. In replacing your drinks, you gradually lose the taste for the unhealthy ones till they are eliminated from your drink options.

Although water is good, many people still do not drink as they should. Perhaps the characteristic of being without taste has contributed largely to this. To help with that, add a bit of flavour to your water. This can be easily done with cucumber, lemon, or fresh ginger. Other options that have been seen to aid drinking are to take it as tea, decide on what teabags you would be taking, or nutritionally certified water flavours sold in supermarkets that can be added to your drinking water. Either of these options would be good for a trial, particularly for those with difficulties drinking water. Final tips on this include getting a fancy bottle with measurements to see how much water is taken and always going around with water to drink. It subtly serves as a reminder to stay well hydrated and a form of environmental conditioning to aid increased fluid intake.

Having stated that, I believe you now see that EATING TO WEALTH is a journey of baby steps. Start practicing already. Go ahead and take a sip!

Question

1.   Do you take enough water daily?

2.   What can you do to improve your daily fluid intake?

3.   What drinks do you need to reduce taking, if any?

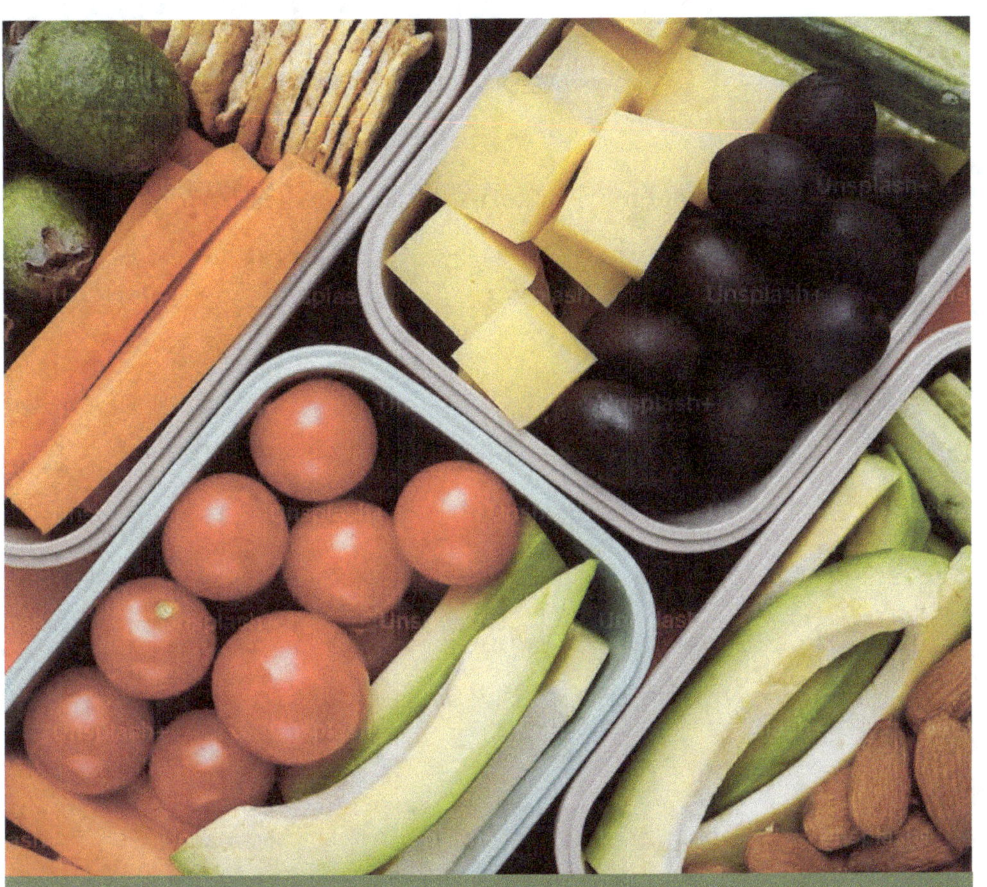

BONUS:
35 SNACK OPTIONS TO CONSIDER

1. **Popcorns**: Popcorns serve as a healthy snack option that can either be made at home or purchased. Less-sweetened/salted popcorns are a better choice.

2. **Plantain chips**: These are also good options to have as snacks in controlled measures.

3. **Guacamole**: Let's call it avocado dip. It has different recipes but is often a mix of avocado with tomatoes, black pepper, onions, spices, and anything you desire. Makes for a filling snack and a sumptuous dip.

4. **Sweet potato/Plantain chips and guacamole**: Either of these go well with guacamole, so you should try it.

5. **Garden eggs and nut butter**: This is a snack you have probably had or encountered someone eating. Either the white or green garden eggs,

eaten alongside the locally made or store-bought nut or peanut butter.

6. **Bananas and nuts**: Bananas are a healthy source of potassium, fiber, and vitamins like vitamin C. They can be taken alone or with groundnuts.

7. **Fruit salad**: This is a really flexible combination of mixed fruits that makes for a good go-to snack you didn't know you needed.

8. **Trail mix**: This is simply having groundnut, almond nuts, cashew nuts, raisins, pistachio, etc., in a bowl together to be munched on.

9. **Dried fruits**: Dried fruits are increasingly becoming available in local stores and online. They are quite filling, too, due to their increased fiber content.

10. **Yoghurt**: Plain or sweetened yoghurt taken alone or as parfait can make good snack options.

11.   **Apples:** An apple a day keeps the Doctors away. Snack as you may!

12.   **Apples and nuts/ peanut butter**: Instead of having the apples alone, take them with peanut or almond butter.

13.   **Hard-boiled eggs**: Eggs are a good option because they contain a whole lot of nutrients in them (*except Vitamin C*). Having a whole egg in between meals is a good idea.

14.   **Dark chocolate**: Ever heard of dark chocolates contributing to heart health? You may want to be selective with chocolates when shopping next. Watch the portions too.

15.   **Carrot cake**: Cakes are yummy and are widely available in different flavours. Getting a slice to go with a cup of tea is a good mid-day snack.

16. **Carrot sticks**: Their crunchiness, colour, taste, and health benefits make them a great snack.

17. **Granola bars**: Healthy replacements for sugar-laced munchies. Contains oats, nuts, and dried fruits.

18. **Kuli kuli**: A common West African snack made from groundnuts. Comes in cylindrical strips, round or flattened shapes, and is now readily found in stores.

19. **Coconut chips**: May be coated in sugar, and spices, or served plain. A very crunchy addition to parfaits.

20. **Well-made pies**: Chicken/Meat pie - The addition of veggies, chicken/minced meat, and Irish potato to the dough base makes this a good snack option. Only remember not to have too much of it.

21.   **Boiled groundnuts**: These nutrient-dense snacks are quite something! Beware - They can be a bit addictive.

22.   **Cashew nuts**: Cashew nuts are filling and rich in nutrients. They are also considered as part of healthy fat options.

23.   **Smoothies**: These are a great way to achieve your fruit servings as it is easier to consume when in blended form. You'd do well to search out different recipes.

24.   **Corn (boiled/roasted) and purple yam**: A lightweight delicacy popularly called *corn and ube in Nigeria*.

25.   **Water yam fritters**: popularly known as Ojojo. Is usually made from grating water yam and then frying. This, like akara (bean cake), can also be taken as a meal or a snack. Protein options like crayfish or shrimp can be added to the mix.

26. **Almond nuts:** Can be enjoyed alone or alongside other nut types. It can also be processed into milk.

27. **Akara (bean cake)**: Enjoy this as a meal or a side dish. This is often made with black-eyed beans or lentils.

28. **Walnuts**: A rare but nutrient-packed option.

29. **Biscuits**: To avoid naming brands, cracker biscuits or less sweetened biscuits are generally safe for consumption but feel free to try other biscuits in moderation and do so occasionally.

30. **Roasted plantain and nuts**: Bole/boli refers to roasted plantain that you then eat with nuts. Some take this with fish sauce or as barbecue.

31. **Dates:** Dates contain a good amount of vitamins and fiber and are also processed into sugar i.e. the

powdered form, which can be substituted for regular sugar. Dates powder is available in stores.

32.   **Egg roll**: Although, the egg in the roll makes this a go-to option for you, avoid rolls that have a heavy or thick dough.

33.   **Scotch eggs**: Similar to the egg roll but with a different taste and texture.

34.   **Whole fruits**: you cannot go wrong with taking fruits except if consumed excessively (*reference daily servings required*). Cucumbers, watermelon, pineapples, mangoes, pawpaw, and many others are all good fruits that make for healthy snack options.

35.   **Soya milk**: Some brands have been able to make this available in different flavours and they serve as good protein sources. Now you have a variety to choose from.

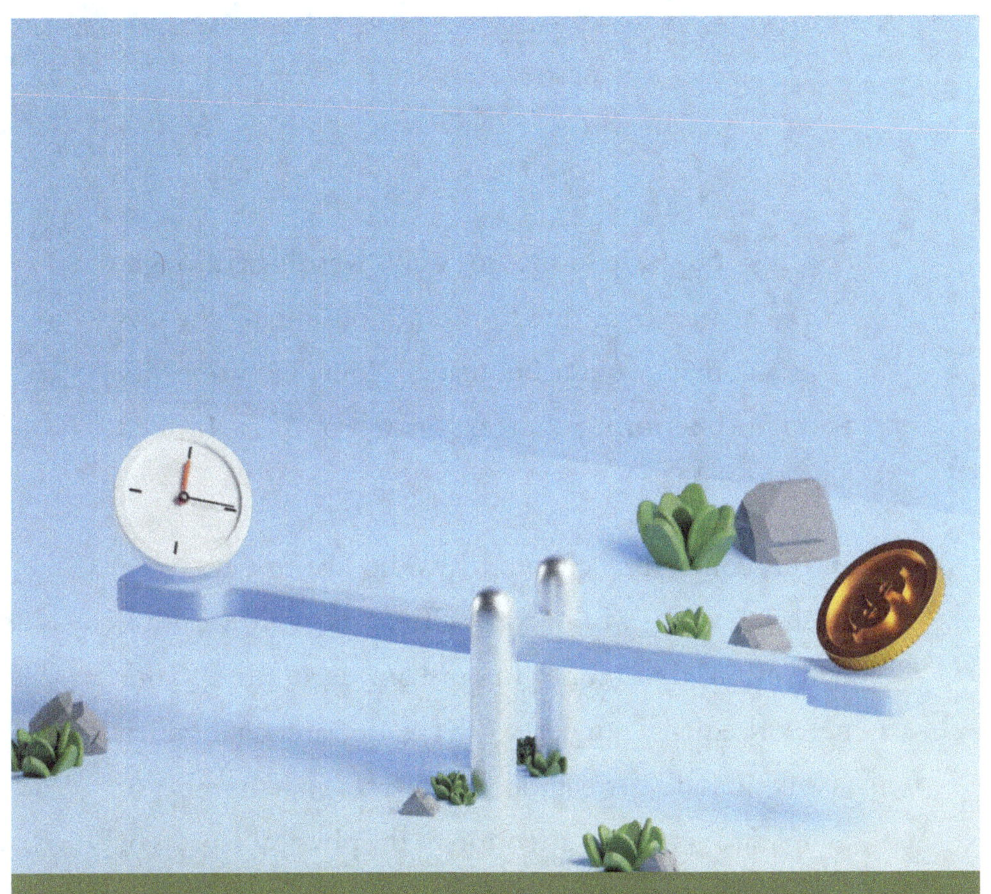

YOUR WEALTH ZONE

You have done so well! Reading through, answering questions, and considering changes that would be made. Your intentionality toward becoming better with food is indeed commendable.

In this concluding chapter, I would like to draw your attention to the wealth zone. Often, the word wealth is tied or linked to money in our bank accounts or 'your network equals your net worth', i.e., social capital, which is very fine and correct too. However, a good number of people are yet to pay attention to the physical aspects of our wealth.

Wealth is commonly classified into four areas as seen below:

- **Physical wealth** - refers to how healthy you are physically and mentally.

- **Time wealth** - the freedom to choose what you want to do when you want to.

- **Social wealth** - where our social capital lies, i.e., the meaningful relationships we build.

- **Financial wealth** - or financial freedom, which most people are familiar with.

Your health is possibly the most important part of your wealth type and serves as the foundation on which every other wealth block is built. Only a healthy person can create and utilize the other aspects of wealth optimally. Moreso, what is the point of making so much financial wealth only to spend it on an ailment that could have been prevented from happening?

More often than not, the foods we eat contribute to the build-up of diseases in the body. Data from the World Health Organisation shows that an unhealthy diet is one of the major contributory factors to diseases like Cancer, heart disease, liver problems, etc. Many of them are tied to what we eat or do not eat as we ought to.

As a young person reading this, there is no need to delay your decision to make necessary adjustments till you are much older. It would be great to build the proper habits now. As a middle-aged or elderly person, it is not too late to change. With the knowledge you have gained here and will continue to seek and make use of, I encourage you to make healthy food choices a habit.

There is so much we can do to aid our physical wealth, and as a Medical Doctor, I can tell you for sure that **prevention is ALWAYS better than cure**. However, if there are medical conditions you are currently being managed for, as you use your medications, still do well to eat right.

You have come this far, and here are my concluding words from John the Beloved to you:

"Beloved friend, I pray that you are prospering in every way and that you continually enjoy good health, just as your soul is prospering."

(**3 John 1:2**, The Passions Translation (TPT) of the Holy Bible.)

Eat to Wealth and not to death.

Cheers to Healthy living!

FREQUENTLY ASKED QUESTIONS (FAQs)

1. Now that I have read all this, where do I really start?

A: That is simple. The rule is to always start with what you have or where you are and then make improvements. Different ideas will come up in your mind now that you are conscious of eating healthily. Take steps on them.

For a systematic approach, you may decide to itemize the areas you want to work on and put a timeframe for each one, but if that will overwhelm you, simply start with what you can now, e.g., drinking more water or adding more vegetables to your meals, and then continue to adjust gradually.

2.   Is eating healthy expensive?

A: When considering cost, put into consideration the long-term financial benefits attached to eating healthy, and you will realize it saves you resources that would have gone towards avoidable medical bills.

Also, you might want to identify what cost means in your case too.

Time cost? Delegate or outsource. Financial cost? Purchase items in bulk or source from local vendors/farm stores.

3.   What is next after the three-week plan?

A: You either recreate yours, selecting food items from the different food groups and classes, or simply shuffle the weekly meal plans here. You now have the consciousness to eat healthily, so build on that.

4.   Are there foods I should stay away from?

A: While it is advised not to label foods as good or bad, there are foods you should have more of and those you should have less of. The more processed a food, the less of it you should have. Consider the same with your cooking ingredients as well.

5.   How else can I get more resources or continue the journey to healthy living?

A: Follow the Instagram page @eatingtowealth or send an email to eatingtowealth@gmail.com for more inquiries.